# The BDSM Playbook

51 Ready-Made BDSM Scenes for Hot, Kindy & Intense Plays

Elizabeth Cramer

Copyright© 2017 by Elizabeth Cramer

# The BDSM Playbook

Copyright© 2017 Elizabeth Cramer
All Rights Reserved.

Warning: The unauthorized reproduction or distribution of this copyrighted work is illegal. No part of this book may be scanned, uploaded or distributed via internet or other means, electronic or print without the author's permission. Criminal copyright infringement without monetary gain is investigated by the FBI and is punishable by up to 5 years in federal prison and a fine of $250,000. (http://www.fbi.gov/ipr/). Please purchase only authorized electronic or print editions and do not participate in or encourage the electronic piracy of copyrighted material.

Publisher: Living Plus Healthy Publishing

ISBN-13: 978-1548714529

ISBN-10: 1548714526

## Disclaimer

The Publisher has strived to be as accurate and complete as possible in the creation of this book. While all attempts have been made to verify information provided in this publication, the Publisher assumes no responsibility for errors, omissions, or contrary interpretation of the subject matter herein. Any perceived slights of specific persons, peoples, or organizations are unintentional.

This book is not intended for use as a source of legal, business, accounting or financial advice. All readers are advised to seek services of competent professionals in the legal, business, accounting, and finance fields.

The information in this book is not intended or implied to be a substitute for professional medical advice, diagnosis or treatment. All content contained in this book is for general information purposes only. Always consult your healthcare provider before carrying on any health program.

# Table of Contents

Introduction ......................................................... 3

Sexual Scenarios for Beginners .......................... 5

Nonsexual Scenarios for Beginners ................. 19

Sexual Scenarios Establishing Trust ............... 29

Nonsexual Scenarios Establishing Trust ....... 43

Conclusion ........................................................ 99

Other Books by Elizabeth Cramer ................ 100

# Introduction

In BDSM lifestyle, a lot of couples and individuals complain that although they understand the dynamic and emotion, they still have trouble coming up with scenes to try. Maybe they feel silly reenacting movies or porn or just draw a blank when asked for suggestions. This is why it's helpful to use a BDSM workbook or playbook, containing a number of scenes for both sexual and nonsexual game play.

In this book, we're going to review 51 scenes that you can try and adapt to your own lifestyle and routine. They are separated into categories of Beginners (sexual and nonsexual), Earning Trust, and Extreme Power Plays. These scenes will teach you characters, behaviors and thinking patterns that will help you forget yourself and start thinking in terms of finishing scenes and following your "natural" emotions.

They will also help you to let go of all inhibitions and give yourself to the scene, whether as a Dom or sub. For some scenes we also covered ideas for adding additional players into the mix, should you reach that level.

However, understand that all of the scenes are highly malleable to your own purposes. You can adapt the sexual scenes into nonsexual behavior; for example, substituting sex with spanking, ice play, heat play, needle play, electroshock, flogging or bondage. You can also turn the nonsexual routines into sexual, should you reach that point where you want both.

You can also add more players and delegate responsibility with multiple Doms or bring other subs into the scene to give the Dom even more power and enjoyment. It's better to personalize each of these scenarios to your own preferences, which you will discuss in dialog during the negotiation phase. Write out a contract, as always, just to make sure no one is surprised or hurt by the scenario or what happens in it. BDSM is all about open communication.

Once you try these 51 BDSM scenes, you will be an advanced player capable of creating even more captivating ideas!

# Sexual Scenarios for Beginners

*These scenarios are among the easiest to create and improvise to, especially for beginners. While you get used to the dynamic and new territory, you can explore these light-hearted scenarios without much pressure. Try them a few times before exploring the more taboo and exciting scenarios just to make sure you got the hang of it.*

## 1. The Dominant Husband and his Wife

**The Setting:** This is such an easy scenario to start with, that many people actually live this lifestyle in real life! The husband is the bread winner so he gets to decide what his wife does, where and when, micromanaging her in every respect—especially the bedroom. He decides after a good meal and good evening, he wants sex. The wife is shy as always, so he takes the lead in telling her what he wants.

**Why It Works:** Many men today are feminist-minded, at least to the extent that they want to please women and not behave like a chauvinist. However, sometimes they are so well behaved they forget what a turn on it can be for a woman to be sexually dominant and to come up with most of the bedroom routine. This guy is a little selfish but he's macho and confident and that makes the scenario hot.

**How to Make It Good:** Don't act too much like yourself. Try to let your wife or girlfriend see a new side of you, one that knows what he wants and isn't ashamed to demand it. Use a different voice or a different set of clothes to help immerse yourself in the character. Be selfish and take what you want from her body.

**The Climax:** You can have fun with this, as the husband can just finish up and leave the bed, letting the wife feel violated in a good way.

**Props:** Perhaps jeans and an old "wife beater" T-shirt.

**Where?:** A bedroom or a hotel, or better yet a vacation house. Somewhere that's unfamiliar.

**Variant:** You don't have to be married. He can be the oafish "Stanley Kowalski", a brute who calls the girl on their mutual attraction and goes in for a rough kiss.

### 2. Hollywood Starlet and the Cab Driver

**The Setting:** This setting is the reverse of the Dominant Husband and allows the woman to be dominant, sexual and tell the "cab driver" exactly how she wants it. The starlet starts flirting with the man, instantly sensing that he's shy but very attracted to her. She gets to tell him how she likes it, while he tries halfheartedly to resist, fearing for his job. But in the end, he always goes for it.

**Why It Works:** Notice that the man is not obligated to do what she says, but finds it difficult to resist her smoldering sexuality. He knows it's dangerous but still has a hard time saying no. So even though the woman is in control and dominant sexually, she still has to persuade the man to give into temptation.

**How to Make It Good:** The starlet knows what she wants and will tell the man what to do to please her, rather than expecting him to know how to do it. She is very demanding. This gives women the same opportunity to be dominant like in the previous scenario, for men.

**The Climax:** The movie starlet, much like the dominant husband, enjoys just using the limo driver sexually and dismissing him.

**Props:** The starlet should get all dolled up like somebody's favorite movie star. The limo driver should be dressed in a suit.

**Where?:** Start in the car, either a rental limo or your own. End in a hotel or bedroom.

**Variant:** Instead of a Hollywood star, she could be a rich heiress or powerful CEO, and he could be anything from a pool boy or a fan of the movie star.

## 3. The Charming Seducer and the Innocent Youth

**The Setting:** There is always something very exciting about an older and experienced lover seducing someone younger who is curious and "green" when it comes to sexuality. Sometimes we imagine these scenarios in terms of family, as in "my girlfriend's mom" or "my boyfriend's older brother", or among strangers; "The Hollywood Actor seduces a young waitress" or "The sexy cougar preys upon a naïve young gardener." You can use one of these or make your own unique scenario, but the dynamic is always the same: experience seducing innocence.

**Why It Works:** The attractiveness of an older lover is usually because we as individuals associate guilt when it comes to asking or influencing another person for sex. Therefore, if we are "seduced" rather than willfully try to have sex with someone, we can indulge ourselves without reluctance. The older lover takes all responsibility for the relationship. Plus, the younger lover gets experience in trying new things he/she never tried before.

**How to Make It Good:** Part of the fun is in saying no, at least at first. However, since the older lover is so charming, he eventually seduces the younger one into doing something scandalous.

**The Climax:** The younger lover always feels a little ashamed that she went this far. But he/she cannot resist the other one's charms.

**Props:** Add some wine to the scenario, since the younger lover always seems to make more mistakes when slightly intoxicated.

**Where?:** Anywhere, perhaps even in a secluded public place. Just don't get caught!

**Variant:** It always helps to know that the young lover's family hates the experienced lover. So work that that scenario in for sparks.

## 4. The Hot Teacher and Student

**The Setting:** The Hot Teacher (male or female) is the Dominant and takes advantage of the student. This scenario is similar to the previous one but with one significant difference. There is a clear power mismatch, which in the real world, is immoral. The teacher doesn't simply seduce the student, but overpowers her intellectually. He doesn't really give the student much of a choice to resist. The teacher is an authority figure and thus both seduces and intimidates the student into improper activity.

**Why It Works:** Another scenario about guilt. The student is literally "forced" to go along with the teacher's wishes, since objecting to his advances would jeopardize grades and future career paths. The student commits no wrong, since all responsibility lies with the teacher. Yet the student can still secretly enjoy being sexually exploited.

**How to Make It Good:** The teacher should not give the student a choice, like in the other scenarios. The teacher gloats about his or her power, saying that in order to pass a test or not fail, (or not tell the parents) the student must cooperate.

**The Climax:** The teacher wants the illicit relationship to continue and so tells the student that she has special reason to see them again.

**Props:** Anything that can class up the room, like a chalkboard, a desk or a locked room. The teacher should dress up, establishing authority compared to the casually dressed student.

**Where?:** If you have access to an office fixing it up like a classroom could be fun.

**Variant:** Although the student is usually excited to indulge the teacher, removing the appearance of consent can have its own fun. The student may not like what's happening but has no choice but to service the teacher...leading to an erotic taboo of ambivalent emotions.

### 5. The Boss and the Secretary

**The Setting:** This is another power trip scenario involving a different type of authority figure. Whereas the student has no choice but to follow the teacher, the secretary always has a choice to walk away. The game is, that she cannot afford to lose her job. She has several bills due and depends on this job. The boss knows this and exploits the secretary sexually.

**Why It Works:** Another example of control. The boss demands that the employee entertain him or risk losing the much needed job. In the real world people go out of their way to avoid sexual harassment lawsuits and so even consensual flirting is a very dangerous idea. This is a way to have fun with it in an exaggerated fantasy world.

**How to Make It Good:** Make the boss a little naughty and not overly concerned about the employee's welfare. A good boss would not ask for sexual favors. An evil boss would. He may even remind the secretary why she needs this job; medical bills, late rent, car payments, etc.

**The Climax:** After the boss climaxes, work always continues as usual, and the lover doesn't really get any "special favors" besides getting to keep her job.

**Props:** Make one of your rooms to be an office with a desk, laptop and chairs...and be sure to use the desk!

**Where?:** This can be done at home, your own office, or a hotel business room.

**Variant:** Instead of the boss exploiting the employee, another twist is that the employee is so desperate to keep the job (after making a mistake or being laid off) that he or she offers sex in return for not being fired.

## 6. The Police Officer and the Motorist

**The Setting:** The police officer is the dominant in this scenario and can bully the motorist however he or she wants. In this scenario, the sub is terrified of going to jail and facing arrest and so is willing to do anything to get out of legal punishment.

**Why It Works:** Another scenario where angering the Dom is the erotic element, not just the excitement of sex. The Dom must stay in character and be commanding, treating the sub like a criminal and demanding, not asking, sexual favors in return for letting them go. This is an exaggeration of what everyone fears in the real world: a corrupt cop, who is open to bribes.

**How to Make It Good:** Make the crime fairly realistic, like being busted for marijuana, a speeding ticket, a warrant for arrest, or something that would be intimidating. You could even make it a major crime like drug dealing, suspicion of fraud or murder, or something like that.

**The Climax:** The police officer is not sentimental or cuddly and will dismiss the suspect after the deed is done. (This doesn't count as the "aftermath" of a BDSM scene...only the end of the "scene" itself)

**Props:** Definitely rent or buy a police officer's uniform, even if it's fake. Handcuffs anyone? Handcuffs are good to experiment with but you might want to take them off when you get into the nitty-gritty, since they tend to hurt. For your first time being tied up, consider restraints with some scenarios below.

**Where?:** It works better to actually stop your partner out in public and make initial contact that way. From there you can take them home or to a hotel and "book" them before you discuss a negotiation.

**Variant:** If the sub likes a man or woman in uniform, the cop can be incarnated into a sergeant intimidating a cadet instead.

## 7. The John and the Prostitute

**The Setting:** The John (or Jane) seeks a prostitute for a purely sexual relationship. He makes demands from the prostitute, and she is not really in a position to refuse. They exchange money when the act is finished.

**Why It Works:** This gives both partners the opportunity to experiment sexually, segregating sex from love and romance. They negotiate for the services they want, negotiating from the outset. This is a good way to introduce new foreplay into the routine, or simply to spice up regular sexual routines.

**How to Make It Good:** Make up new names for each other and act contrary to your natural personality. This is not really about you pretending to be a prostitute or John. It's about exploring a taboo, if you and your partner were somebody else entirely. What would you do? How would you act?

**The Climax:** Exchange money for services, as is the custom. (Although a smart working girl knows to charge upfront)

**Props:** Sexy and sultry clothing, usually the opposite of what a woman usually thinks is sexy...something more outrageous and revealing.

**Where?:** Definitely a hotel, somewhere away from home. Getaway vacations may be ideal.

**Variant:** You can make the John shy or dominant, each for a different effect. Like the other scenarios this one thrives on power exchange. The shy boy is taken by the older lover, or the older man gets to dominate the young innocent.

# Nonsexual Scenarios for Beginners

*Many BDSM players do not actually want sex, or may only occasionally want sex, but prefer a lot more in the way of actual punishment and other BDSM activity. These scenarios are exclusively for partners who want to experiment with beginning punishment scenarios but not actually cross a line.*

## 8. Nanny and the Bad Kid

**The Setting:** Nanny can be either sex, as can the naughty boy or girl. This is not necessarily an age play; the age can be irrelevant or without any concrete details. All that you know is that the Nanny must punish the Bad Boy or Girl for what they've done. Because this is nonsexual, any sexual innuendos the Bad Kid addresses are reason for further punishment from the strict Nanny.

**Why It Works:** This is an introduction to punishment without going in too deep. The Nanny punished the Bad Boy with the intent of correcting his bad behavior. Nothing about this scenario is sexual and yet it may be very exciting to experience, whether you want sex or not. Feeling punishment and getting physically punished for your mistakes is a new sense of emotional release you may not have experienced.

**How to Make It Good:** Talk to the sub while disciplining her. Like a good parent, make sure she understands the punishment. Talk about the spanking, how it feels, how it hurts, as if you were talking during sex. Make it intense. Rather than talking about sexual things ("You're a slut! You like when I fuck you?"), instead convert it to spanking talk. ("You're a bad boy. You deserve a spanking. You will be spanked until you cooperate.")

**The Climax:** After the punishment is given the Nanny assures the Bad Kid that he is still loved but that punishment was necessary to help him correct his behavior. Some touching and hugging might be done here.

**Props:** Choose a simple form of punishment at first, such as a hand spanking or even a paddle from school. You can also use a small whip or flogger, but avoid anything too intense for now.

**Where?:** Any location but a hotel is very discreet and allows you to let go more than a home.

**Variant:** A teacher and student relationship can work here, as teachers used to actually spank kids a long time ago and there usually wasn't anything sexual about it.

## 9. The Kidnapper and the Hostage

**The Setting:** While this may sound sexual, for this particular scene it is not. Rather, the Kidnapper just has the task of tying the hostage up and awaiting further instructions. The joy here is being tired up, powerless and feeling vulnerable. The kidnapper can stare and touch when necessary, but he is not to sexually torment the sub in this scenario.

**Why It Works:** This is a beginner's game, just to give both participants the feeling of domination and submission. While later games will experiment with sex, this is all about anticipation and vulnerability. The Kidnapper could take advantage of the sub, but chooses not to. The feeling is still there and for a beginner, that's enough to work with. The sub shifting around and gasping will be a turn on for both partners.

**How to Make It Good:** Make sure the Dom knows how to tie a rope or operate the tying mechanism, to a professional level. This exercise can be dangerous if he doesn't know about proper tying technique and accidentally hurts the sub. Once the sub is tied she can resist or try to squeeze out of the bondage gear. But she should not be able to escape.

**The Climax:** The scene ends when the Kidnapper talks to the Hostage's family and gets the ransom money paid.

**Props:** Rope, restraints, handcuffs, straightjackets, wrap, etc.

**Where?:** Any location but a hotel is more thrilling.

**Variant:** For a different flavor, you can change the Kidnapper's motivation to revenge rather than ransom money. Maybe he's getting her back for a business swindle.

## 10. Drill Sergeant and New Cadet

**The Setting:** The drill sergeant explains to the cadet the training at hand and why it must be done for the good of the country. The drill sergeant is very stern, loud and inconsiderate of the cadet's feelings. Therefore he can be harsh but only pushes the cadet towards self-improvement.

**Why It Works:** The drill sergeant barking orders to the new cadet has the feeling of "duty", of patriotic responsibility, not sexual domination. Therefore, everything you do, however kinky or taboo you decide on making it, will be in the spirit of survival and for military training. If you have a military romance fantasy or just respect the uniform this may be a good non-sexual scenario that will get you excited about training.

**How to Make It Good:** Make it somewhat convincing, as if the sergeant is only training the cadet so that he will know how to respond to torture from enemy agents in the future. Explain how all this punishment will help to toughen the sub up.

**The Climax:** The drill sergeant, while tough, does believe in rewarding a cadet's behavior when he is obedient. But again, he only gives very little love, mostly manly appreciation and encouragement for a job well done.

**Props:** This would be good for exploring nonsexual BDSM practices, whether spanking, hot wax or ice play, and other physical stimuli.

**Where?:** Any location preferably away from home.

**Variant:** You may choose to change the dynamic in this scenario according to desired effect; does the drill sergeant want you to cooperate and willfully take the punishment or is the mission "Show no pain?" You can vary the effect with each round, as the trainer strengthens the sub in different ways each time.

### 11. Personal Trainer Gone Mad

**The Setting:** The personal trainer is going above and beyond the duties explained. Whereas he should be teaching the client to lose weight or get fit, he is instructing her to do some rather weird practices that we can only assume is for his own evil pleasure. For example, the personal trainer could pretend as if spanking a client, or wax/ice play, or causing minor pain in another way is all part of the "no pain no gain" workout routine. The sub is suspicious as to how these practices relate to physical training…but he orders her to not ask questions and undermine his judgment.

**Why It Works:** This can be sexual or entirely nonsexual, with the personal trainer requested invasive information, touching or punishing the sub in unusual ways not related to a work out, or hooking her up to a special pain/pleasure machine instead of a treadmill.

**How to Make It Good:** The personal trainer stays in character, always pretending that this is just an extended workout. He can't admit he is perverted because he has his reputation to consider. But he exploits the naiveté of his sub and instructs her to do vile things for his amusement and her reluctant pleasure.

**The Climax:** The sub will continue to perform the routine, even if it stings or feels erotic, until he tells her to stop. He may give contradictive instructions, such as "Don't enjoy this!" or something to that effect, since he believes he isn't violating any trust. The sub may eventually know she's being exploited but she eventually enjoys the violation. Again, this is one of the few scenarios that doesn't have to be overtly sexual.

**Props:** Workout clothes, stopwatch, towels, tennis shoes, restraints, floggers, and of course water!

**Where?:** Rent a gym or build your own gym room to make it very official looking.

**Variant:** If not a personal trainer, a massage therapists that goes one step too far in subjecting the body to painful/pleasure treatments.

## 12. Martial Arts Master

**The Setting:** A martial arts master is similar to a drill sergeant but teaches the student the esoteric arts. In this case, it would be BDSM pleasure/pain as a way of training the sub in mysticism. Perhaps the Martial Arts Master would instruct her on ways of the samurai, the snake, the ninja, and so on. The point is, the Master can create his own personal course of punishment and dominance/submission without things getting sexual.

**Why It Works:** The student doesn't want to be exploited sexually but trusts the Martial Arts Master to teach her valuable training. This training can hurt and include intense punishment, but the Master Martial Artist usually doesn't crave sexual satisfaction. He is more interested in the punishment and training regimen itself. He wants to teach the student everything he knows, make her suffer but learn most of all.

**How to Make It Good:** Take time to create each lesson. Make it a little confusing at first; for example, a sponge bath, sitting in darkness, or any other foreplay or BDSM related practice. Have the sub do it without asking questions and then at the end of the scene, explain the significance.

**The Climax:** The Martial Arts Master performs the practice until the sub says no more or until a euphoric high occurs. In the beginning, stages may be shorter so the sub can become accustomed to the more punishing routines.

**Props:** Depending on the chosen activity, this may include spanking instruments, restraints, ice cubes or candles, or other objects. A white Karate style suit may also help you get into the mood of respect and attentiveness.

**Where?:** Anywhere.

**Variant:** If you enjoy Harry Potter, Game of Thrones, make it magical training!

# Sexual Scenarios Establishing Trust

*This section returns to sexual scenarios, but with less emphasis on pushing limits and more activities that strengthen trust between Dom and sub. Before a Dom can push the sub to her limits, trust must be established so that the journey is not terrifying but truly exciting.*

*We will also be adding notes at the end for how to really spice things up with a third or fourth party, if that's what you find exciting. However, these are not recommended unless you want to invite others into your relationship. The Third or Fourth Party can always be simulated.*

## 13. The Dom and his Erotic Novelist

**The Setting:** The Dom instructs the sub to write out a taboo fantasy according to his choosing. He purposely uses the sub's soft limits as inspiration, ordering her to develop a detailed story line according to his notes.

**Why It Works:** This allows the sub to confront her forbidden desires in written form. First she is forced to think about the uncomfortable fantasy, which she still finds exciting. Then she must visualize the incident and then write it down.

**How to Make It Good:** The Dom then orders her to read it back. The story can start simple or be a complex plot, if the Dom chooses. But the sub is both exhilarated and nervous at having to confront these issues.

**The Climax:** The Dom finally forces the sub to masturbate to the story, while reading it aloud.

**Props:** A notepad, electronic or handwritten describing the action.

**Where?:** Anywhere, even online or long distance over the phone.

**Variant:** The Dom can give the shy sub an erotic mission: to go out and perform the sexual task he gave her and then tell him about it in detail. Of course, she doesn't actually do it, not in this game, but she can describe the encounter over a phone as if it really happened.

**Multiples:** Either a friend can be brought into watch or can actually read the story the sub wrote while the Dom and sub reenact it.

### 14. Cleopatra and her Slave

**The Setting:** This scenario is similar to a teacher or Hollywood starlet, but the difference is that the Domme woman gets total power. Under this scenario, the slave boy cannot refuse the Queen's amorous intentions. The other option would be death. So the male slave must surrender all power to the Queen and must make peace with whatever sexual or perverted request she gives him.

**Why It Works:** While the slave / sub does ultimately have control over the scene (as always in BDSM) the illusion that he cannot say no can be erotic. This is especially good for subs who are ready to test their soft limits but still have trepidation about trying something new. The Master, in this case, would push the sub's limits slowly and gently, but consistently. With the illusion that the slave cannot say no to the queen, the anticipation will work to your advantage.

**How to Make It Good:** The slave should address Cleopatra or the Queen by her formal title. She is not the slave's equal but far superior and he must acknowledge that. The Queen's intention is to teach the slave that by follower her orders, he will NOT be exposed to terrifying acts or bullying behavior but that the Queen will make it feel good. Only if he listens to her, will he be assured of a favorable outcome. This game will establish trust so don't move too quickly. The more power you wield the more patient you must be.

**The Climax:** The slave must please the Queen in just the way she asked.

**Props:** Queenly or Egyptian garb with the man scantily clad.

**Where?:** A nice hotel or rental home would work well.

**Variant:** If you want the male reverse, have a King dominating a slave girl or concubine.

**Multiples:** A MMF or FFM threesome would also fit this scene.

## 15. The Photographer and the Model

**The Setting:** The photographer wants to do a sexy but tasteful shoot. The photographer is dominant and experienced about taking erotic photos but the sub is shy and has never thought of herself as a sex symbol. The Photographer must be clever about persuading the sub to follow along. Then, he takes a series of photographs (yes, real photos) and develops them showing the sub the result.

**Why It Works:** This scene is not about domination and power—it's about building trust. The sub is scared about how she will look, and this will be true to life if she has body image issues. Therefore, the Dom lovingly persuades her to follow his lead and trust him, that he will pick only the best pictures and poses to make it sexy.

**How to Make It Good:** The photographer should put thought into the poses and pictures. If you enjoy taking photos or photoshopping, have fun with this. Start with G rated pictures and slowly progress to R-rated nudity and even X-rated porn.

**The Climax:** The photo shoot ends and he delivers the pictures. He lovingly reassures her that it's very sexy and she feels beautiful.

**Props:** Buy the sub new lingerie to help her get into character and feel sexy on his command.

**Where?:** A new environment like a hotel or even an outdoor reclusive area where you can get privacy.

**Variant:** The Artist and the work of art is the same principle, except that instead of photographing a lover in the nude, the sub would be drawn.

**Multiples:** The pictures could be given to a third party for evaluation and he/she could praise the sub for the good work.

### 16. The Gent and the Mail Order Bride

**The Setting:** The Gent just bought a mail order bride. She is a virgin and doesn't know how to consummate the marriage. But the Gent will guide her through it and tell her how a good wife behaves. This is not only a sexual scenario but can include non-sexual interactions. This might include cooking a good meal, cleaning the house, doing laundry and wearing exactly what the master demands. Then, after fulfilling these chores, the master tells her what to do sexually, such as touching herself, taking her clothes off and pleasuring him.

**Why It Works:** Introducing nonsexual practices as foreplay to the sexual routine helps to establish trust, as well as exciting sex. The wife playing the innocent and expressing love by way of doing chores is a throwback to another era and also experiments with submission.

**How to Make It Good:** She is not a "good wife" at first but is apprehensive about doing these chores. However, the Dom persuades her to cooperate since he's already bought her as a bride and she needs to follow his lead if she wants a place to live. The sub should assume a different personality than her natural side, or a stereotypical wife. She may even want to take on a new accent!

**The Climax:** Love is the climax here not just sex. The mail order bride falls in love with the Gent by the end of the night and they cuddle in afterglow.

**Props:** Work household chores into the routine and give her a to do list; cooking utensils, laundry, etc.

**Where?:** At home!

**Variant:** If you want switch play, or woman in power scenarios, a mail order husband or "butler" or "manservant" can accommodate a wealthy socialite.

**Multiples:** Two wives or two husbands would be another scenario, as with a religious cult.

### 17. The Billionaire's Auction

**The Setting:** It's not just one billionaire but a number of billionaires bidding on the sub. They can do whatever they want to the sub once the money has been paid. The winner takes her home and does whatever he wants for the entire night. The sub is afraid, and afraid of some creepy billionaires more than others.

**Why It Works:** This is another game of trust since the Billionaire can do whatever he wants sexually or masochistically, even if it scares the sub. Another training and trust game, since the all-powerful billionaire must show the sub that complete submission will only lead to pleasure and protection, not danger or harm. But full trust is required. Naturally, these would only be soft limits and progression would be slow.

**How to Make It Good:** The Dom should play ALL the parts of the perverted billionaires for anticipation. Make one billionaire a complete pervert. Make the other one harsh and cold. Make another one mysterious and another one kind. Half the fun will be in learning which Billionaire gets the girl and what he's going to do to her. Decide in advance by writing down the name of the highest bidding billionaire.

**The Climax:** The billionaire challenges her limits but ultimately earns her trust because she obediently performs his request.

**Props:** Make the sub and Billionaire Dom dress up for a formal occasion.

**Where?:** Preferably somewhere away from home.

**Variant:** Billionaire Domme can order a young man and buy his services just as well.

**Multiples:** Have a real bidding war between the two Doms who offer complete opposite but exciting punishments/rewards. Or, have multiple fearful subs waiting to be chosen by a Dom or Doms by random lottery.

## 18. Mind Controlling Supervillain

**The Setting:** The supervillain can control the sub with his mind, therefore eliminating all control she has over her own behavior. However, he doesn't have to physically do anything. He tells her what to do in great detail and step by step, perhaps even hours in advance. He tells her when to get ready, what to wear, and when she should take her clothes off and get in bed. He starts every new step with "You will" and the sub must be obedient. She doesn't have to enjoy it...but she will do each task because all actions are involuntary.

**Why It Works:** The illusion is of complete submission which requires trust—on both partner's end. He trusts her to remember every last detail and she trusts him not to do anything too cruel. This is still part of the trust building process so the Supervillain will not make any demands too strict or overbearing at first. Rather he will test her soft limits and order her to do his bidding. Not knowing what he will request, but still vowing to do everything will be her duty. She will please him, not by enjoying it necessarily, but by remembering every last detail.

**How to Make It Good:** Don't make the villain too corny. Think of him as more of a strong silent type who has discovered a dangerous secret, one that gives him mental powers over women. All through the process, have the sub "resist" in either voice or just feeling. Let her feel opposed to the act, even though she fulfills it.

**The Climax:** He will order her to make love to him, thus not actually "forcing" her physically. But mentally, he will retain full power over her and exploit her inability to protest. He will reward her for a job well done by releasing the master grip on her mind, freeing her. If she fails to remember every step, he will punish her.

**Props:** Use lingerie, blindfolds, vibrators, lubricant, and other sex toy supplies to give the sub a full list of actions that she must fulfill.

**Where?:** Any location.

**Variant:** Switch the scenario by having a superheroine dominating a criminal in prison.

**Multiples:** Have a third or fourth party watch making the sub even more excited.

## 19. Vampire and Human

**The Setting:** A vampire traps his victim in chains and contemplates whether to drink her blood or kill her. The sub pleads for her life and the Vampire feels attracted to her and then takes her sexually instead.

**Why It Works:** The Vampire is a powerful Dom who is dangerous and mentally powerful. He also carries the illusion of danger, murder and blood sucking.

**How to Make It Good:** If the sub has a vampire or bloodletting fetish, blood capsules or Kool-Aid can be used to make the scene more realistic.

**The Climax:** The session can end with the vampire chomping her and giving her a hickey at the crux of climax.

**Props:** Costumes and Halloween or Gothic décor works wonders for the ambiance.

**Where?:** Preferably a hotel you can decorate to look spooky.

**Variant:** Other popular horror clichés might include shifters. Cutting and blood play are an option if that's a taboo that both partners have.

**Multiples:** Another watching party also dressed as a vampire, or perhaps another innocent hostage forced to watch.

## 20. Internet Stalker and Victim

**The Setting:** In this setting, the sub agrees to be stalked online by a "catfish". The Dom has instructed the sub that he will send someone to her. He doesn't tell her any details nor a time frame but says that once this person contacts her she must do everything he asks. The Do will assume a new name and new online picture. He will know exactly what turns her on. He will seem familiar and yet different. He will eventually make sexual demands which the sub must do. Like cybering in text, or sending sext messages, or sending erotic photos or video. The Stalker may also give her instructions and tell her to turn on the web cam and perform for him.

**Why It Works:** It feels like cheating and yet is not. It also flirts with danger since most women will not want to do what a random Internet stranger demands. However, since the Dom told her to play along, she must show trust in him and obey whatever the stranger says.

**How to Make It Good:** Make the Internet stalker work slowly. He seduces her first, not just makes demands. He entertains her, impresses her and charms her. Then he starts the slow seduction and corruption. Make the new stranger as realistic and different as possible, if you're the Dom. Give her the joy of falling for someone new who seems to know her intimately.

**The Climax:** The Dom will never acknowledge that it's him. He will seduce her into cyber sex, sending erotic photos and video of herself and then just disappear.

**Props:** An online messenger, plenty of fake photos that you can "borrow" from other people, faking social media accounts and the like.

**Variant:** The Dom could also do the same game through email or snail mail.

**Multiples:** If you're comfortable with the idea, enlist a third party to delegate some of the responsibilities. The sub actually does send pictures or texts to a Second Dom at the order of the first.

# Nonsexual Scenarios Establishing Trust

*Once you advance beyond the peripherals and feel the explosive dynamic of dominance and submission, the next stage is establishing trust in a non-sexual but still intimate way. This next section pushes the envelope, but challenges your mind in terms of intimacy without sexual gratification.*

*We will also be adding notes at the end for how to really spice things up with a third or fourth party, if that's what you find exciting. However, these are not recommended unless you want to invite others into your relationship. The Third or Fourth Party can always be simulated.*

## 21. Daddy Punishes Teenager

**The Setting:** We've already done the nanny-parent discipline scenario but this is one step beyond. Spanking doesn't work on rebellious teenagers so you usually have to think of creative ways of punishing them—and the same is true in this scenario. You are either a daddy or some type of parental guardian and you must provide discipline to your teen. This might involve not speaking to them, forcing them to wear something uncomfortable or degrading, or to sit in time out. Another punishment might be taking away a computer or tablet, changing their sleep schedule, or changing the sub's diet to less delicious food. You can also make the sub watch movies she doesn't like. Other creative punishments include making them take a cold shower, cuffing their hands behind their back, or making them stay in a bath for an extended period of time.

**Why It Works:** This is real punishment and nothing builds trust like punishment, apology and affirmation. The sub will experience disappointment and pain but her love for her Dom will be renewed. He will reward her with affection. She will even start to crave more punishment as time goes on, since this usually means the parent showing more love than usual.

**How to Make It Good:** Think in terms of what stresses a person on a daily basis when coming up with punishments. Is there certain work the sub despises or does meeting people make them uncomfortable? This can all be worked into the punishment phase. For the best results, don't punish her randomly. Catch something she's doing without realizing (laughing, not calling you by your title, etc.) and then punish her immediately so she'll associate the negative behavior with punishment and reshape her thinking and actions.

**The Climax:** He holds the sub affectionately and teaches her a lesson on obedience.

**Where?:** At home.

**Variant:** The Mother, Nanny or another female authority figure can do the same in punishing a rebellious teenage boy.

**Multiples:** Mom and dad can both preside over the teen's discipline at the same time.

## 22. The Mentor and the Newbie

**The Setting:** It's time for the Mentor to micromanage the newbie's life, because frankly the newbie can't handle living day by day. The Mentor decides to set a daily schedule for the newbie and to follow each and every command by the hour. The Mentor also decides when the newbie sub can engage in any time of sex or masturbation, (not with him, however), when they shower, eat, exercise and so on. The Mentor also wants the sub to go out into world, although he doesn't trust her to do it alone. He will have more requirements for when she interacts.

**Why It Works:** The Mentor isn't really a "daddy" figure, but a domineering presence who occasionally feels the need to put down the newbie sub, reminding them that they can't do anything right, or anything without the Mentor's help. This is very light humiliation play, but taking it very slow. The intent is not to make the sub feel bad but to feel inadequate of their own power, thus relying on the Mentor just to get through the day.

**How to Make It Good:** Make humiliation part of the trust and non-erotic pain-pleasure emotion. Have the sub address you in "baby talk" so that she can be reminded of her inferiority. She must ask permission to do anything, even if she has to call or email the Dom after session hours. She must follow the Dom Mentor's instructions EVEN when conversing with other people who are unaware of the game. (For example, not looking other people in the eye, talking only to the Mentor Dom)

**The Climax:** If the sub messes up the Mentor should punish her, either as a teen or a child with spanking.

**Where?:** This should be a city-wide game and extend beyond one or two sessions since it involves giving the sub homework.

**Variant:** If you want to give it a more taboo feeling, the Mentor can become a literal parent, mom or dad managing the life of a child, or perhaps an adopted parent if that's more comfortable.

**Multiples:** Good scenario for the Dom training a second Dom.

## 23. The Dom Adopts a Pet

**The Setting:** The Dom has decided to adopt a pet—literally, a nice cat or dog, which will be played by the sub. The sub will literally assume the role of an animal. She will cease talking and instead bark, growl or meow to the Dom when he speaks. Besides that, all she can do is point with her head, or stare at an object, to communicate her needs. Mostly the Dom takes care of all her needs, including eating, sleeping and planning her trips to the bathroom.

**Why It Works:** This not only builds trust and intimacy, but gives the Dom a chance to give the sub lots of affection. He pets the cat / dog and speaks lovingly. However, he also gives strict obedience in telling her when to sit and when to lay down. When she misbehaves he speaks in a lower and more negative tone to correct her. He can also sentence her to time out. This helps improve communication and sensitivity to emotion and faces, since no words are allowed from the sub's mouth.

**How to Make It Good:** Have the sub walk and lie like a four-legged animal. Punish the sub if she breaks character. You can also issue instructions to the sub on licking herself, giving her a bath or walking her (not in public, of course).

**The Climax:** The sub must perform a ritual of the Dom's choosing to go back to being human again.

**Props:** If desired, the sub can sleep or spend time out in a dog house or cat bed, specially made by the Dom. It's also fun to apply whiskers with makeup or dog / cat ears before the game begins.

**Where?:** Around the house.

**Variant:** You can make the sub assume the characteristics of any animal, from snake to pig to cow or horse.

**Multiples:** The Dom allows a second Dom or sub to pet his trained sub as an animal.

Releasing Your Inhibitions: Extreme Power Play

Now that you've tried several BDSM Scenes and have established trust, it's time to intensify those feelings and challenge yourself. All that you've learned thus far in trust exercises is so you can be pushed beyond what is comfortable and into new and exciting territory. These scenarios are uncomfortable but if you have a partner you trust, they can be amazing "taboo" experiences.

We will also be adding notes at the end for how to really spice things up with a third or fourth party, if that's what you find exciting. However, these are not recommended unless you want to invite others into your relationship. The Third or Fourth Party can always be simulated.

### 24. The Interrogator and the Prisoner

**The Setting:** The interrogator is sent into to torture the truth out of the prisoner. This scenario combines sexual and nonsexual BDSM practices into one session. Now that trust is established it's time to lose yourself as you succumb to the sadistic desires of the Interrogator. The Interrogator will do anything necessary to get the Prisoner to talk. From forced sex to vicious spankings or other BDSM pain play, this is going to get intense!

**Why It Works:** This scenario involves surrendering all power and then losing all control to the Dom, who will make it hurt, make it pleasurable and keep the sub on edge. This game is very good at activating the fight or flight adrenaline rush that follows pain / pleasure play, since it is a form of coercion. Reluctant and involuntary passion can follow the session.

**How to Make It Good:** If you really want to make it fun, then the prisoner should not know what the secret is. That way, she can stay realistically in character and claim she doesn't know the piece of information that the Interrogator wants to know. However, the Interrogator knows what that information is...and at some point, the sub figures the mystery out as to who she is, or what she knows.

**The Climax:** Once the sub realizes the "secret" that the Interrogator has given her, she admits it and the torture ceases. But by then, she's had the truth spanked/sexed out of her.

**Props:** Restraints work brilliantly here, as you can work the feeling of helplessness into the torture.

**Where?:** Hotel works best.

**Variant:** You can also continue with the bad cop / innocent victim routine, if you prefer police officers to espionage. Another alternative is to have the sub know the secret and try to have the Dom guess what it is while role playing.

**Multiples:** Two Doms could torture the Prisoner or two Prisoner subs could be tortured by one Dom.

### 25. The Pirate and the Princess

**The Setting:** The pirate is horny, rugged and adheres to no law. The princess is innocent, terrified and beautiful. What will happen when pirates plunders the village? The Pirate takes the pretty princess, kidnaps her and then makes love to her, whether she enjoys it or not.

Of course rape is something terrible in real life, but when you're playing a game with your partner, there is no reason to feel guilt. The guilt attached to this fantasy may even help you to enjoy it all the more so.

**Why It Works:** This is a play scenario that is somewhat outrageous because of the different time era. However, it is among the top taboo fantasies for women. The feeling of being taken advantage of but still enjoying the intensity of sex is intense, because it relieves the woman of responsibility for sexual indiscretion. If she has no choice but to surrender to him, or even fight against him, it's a crime committed against her. But that makes the feeling of violation, not to mention endorphin release from the struggle, very pleasurable.

**How to Make It Good:** The princess should resist until the very end, fighting him with her arms and legs, but ultimately dominated by his strength. She also objects with her words and tone of voice, occasionally screaming for help.

**The Climax:** The pirate finishes the job and makes the princess his bride. Of course, by the climax she's very much enjoying it.

**Props:** The more disposable clothing the princess can wear the better. Renaissance dress or mock party costumes are great, but in the end, you do want something the pirate can tear off in violent lust.

**Where?:** Definitely somewhere other than home. While outdoors vacation homes would be fun, don't do this type of play in a public place!

**Variant:** You can also make it a robber or high school jock, if you don't want to dress up and make it feel modern.

**Multiples:** The Dom can enlist a Second Dom for holding down the sub, or could violate two sub Princesses.

## 26. The Anonymous Attacker and Victim

**The Setting:** The anonymous attacker carjacks the victim on her way home. He wears a mask so she can't identify him. He takes her to a hotel and blindfolds her. He ties her up. Then he takes his time stripping her and having forced sex with her.

**Why It Works:** It gives you a realistic feeling of rape play and causes strange feelings unlike any other scenario, because of the realism.

**How to Make It Good:** The sub may feel panic so it is very important to have a "password" to let her know that the same Dom is really kidnapping her and everything is still a game. Because the sub may feel that she is really being raped by a stranger at some point, since she cannot see the Dom's face at any time. Using this password is important to maintain trust, and let her know that you have it under control, even in this outrageous scenario.

**The Climax:** When he finishes, he leaves and never reveals his face. He leaves after he finishes. She leaves. She is too ashamed to tell anyone what happened. Or, she tells the husband she was violated and he consoles her.

**Props:** A fake weapon works well and definitely a mask for the Dom, while carjacking her, and then a blindfold for the victim so she can't see the Dom's face. Wear a thick black shirt, black pants, leather gloves and full faced mask.

**Where?:** A car and then a hotel.

**Variant:** Instead of carjacking you can have an arrangement where she dresses in lingerie at a certain time and leaves the door opened. The Dom comes home from work and takes her, while holding a weapon. He keeps the mask on and warns her not to look at him. You could also "knock her out" and continue violating her.

**Multiples:** The Dom can train a second Dom to take the sub, provided the sub is aware of someone else intervening. However, it's up to them to determine if she has to meet the Second Dom in person first.

## 27. The Anonymous Visitor and Victim

**The Setting:** Another variation on the former scenario is for the Dom to have the sub tied up and blindfolded and then leave the house. Later, he returns wearing a mask and suit, and bringing toys. He has sex with her and then leaves. She has no idea who just did that to her but assumes it was her Dom.

**Why It Works:** A rush of sex with a stranger, even though it's completely safe and between two committed partners. The Dom gives her the illusion that he is leaving her vulnerable. He may even tell her that it's NOT going to be him but a friend or a stranger he arranged. She will feel the rush of not knowing but will rely on trust.

**How to Make It Good:** The Dom should do his best to distort his face and body and even penis if possible so that she can't be sure if the Dom is making love to her or a stranger. He should avoid speaking while he pleasures her.

**The Climax:** The Dom returns but never speaks of it, nor does she. She wondered for a moment if that was really him.

**Props:** Vibrators and dildos are best, as well as nipple clamps.

**Where?:** Hotel or home.

**Variant:** The Dom can leave her untied but simply crawl into her bedroom and give her oral sex under the blankets. Then He leaves and the sub wonders if it was really him or not. Another variant is for the burglar to break in but the wife (Domme) to catch him in mid-act and then blackmail him into sex.

**Multiples:** The Dom can train a second Dom to take the sub, provided the sub is aware of someone else intervening.

### 28. Step Parent and Son / Daughter

**The Setting:** This is another coercion play, involving light incest or step parent relationships. It is similar to a teacher roleplay but combines punishment and sex, as the step parent will intimidate and "force" the stepson or daughter to go along with their wishes. The stepson or daughter will not feel right about the encounter but will be ordered by the step parent to go through with it.

**Why It Works:** A lot of people have taboo fantasies about their parents or a parental figure coercing them into sex. They don't want to take the risk of finding a sexual partner...they want to be "forced", "ordered" to go to bed with somebody. They resist, but ultimately go along with it because the stepparent will threaten them if necessary to get what he or she wants.

**How to Make It Good:** Use cutesy names like mommy, daddy, mom, dad, and so on. The stepson or daughter should voice their objections, but the step parent must rationalize why this is OK. Use threats and intimidations, such as telling on the stepson / daughter, throwing a tantrum, crying, threatening to cut them off from inheritance money, and so on.

**The Climax:** Either way: the step parent can reassure the stepson or daughter that it's their dirty little secret, or the parent can be blame the whole thing on the stepson or daughter and claim "you made me do this!"

**Where?:** The home is fine.

**Variant:** Brother-sister or aunt / uncle scenarios could also work.

## 29. The Bully and the Cheating Wife

**The Setting:** A similar scenario to what we've done before, except that a strong Dom is forcing a weaker sub, who is married to someone else, cheat with him. She feels extremely guilty but succumbs to his rough and dominant nature, orgasming reluctantly. Her husband is kind and gentle, her bully is very sexual and loveless. But she is torn between two types of lovers.

**Why It Works:** Cheating is a taboo in real life so it makes sense that two faithful lovers would enjoy toying with the notion in private fantasies. It allows you to vicariously experience infidelity without actually hurting your partner. Of course, the sub or wife gets the benefit of being "forced" so she doesn't feel as if she is being slutty or whorish in reaching out to him…the man is simply making her submit against her will.

**How to Make It Good:** Both Dom and sub can "act", and become someone opposite their normal personalities. Experiment with a different way of talking and thinking. Think selfishly if you are the Dom and think like a weak wife if you are the sub. At first the girl SLAPS him…but that only makes him want her more. The sub can't help but submit to a dominant man even if means hurting the family at home.

**The Climax:** The Dom has sex with her and she feels guilty. But he reminds her that anytime he wants her he can have her. She is his sexual slave, whether she likes it or not.

**Props:** Clothes the Dom can rip off work. The wife can pretend she is talking to her husband while having sex with her bully.

**Where?:** Home or a hotel. Even the home can be fun, since you can "cheat" in your partner's bedroom and feel a naughty thrill.

**Variant:** Not only can you play with the male/female reversal, but you can also change the character to someone's mom or dad. Taking advantage of any one "nice", by being a bully and taking what you want, is the dynamic at work.

**Multiples:** Another Dom or sub could pretend to be the cuckolded party and could leave the room or exit the home, just in time, pretending to be a clueless husband.

## 30. The Blackmailer and the Innocent

**The Setting:** A blackmailer Dom has decided to force the sub into a psychosexual relationship. The sub may be a wife, mother, sister, friend, stranger, or co-worker. (Or the male equivalent) She doesn't want this relationship but the Dom is threatening to tell everybody he knows her dirty little secret. It may be an affair she had, erotic pictures she took, a secret sex tape, or even a non-sexual sin, such as lying in business or lying to the court. The blackmailer has an obligation to turn the innocent in…but he instead chooses to force her into sexual relations.

**Why It Works:** It's the kind of thing that gets banned since blackmail is highly illegal. But it still makes for a hot BDSM scene. The sub feels a new shade of "coercion"; this time, she doesn't want to do it but chooses to go along with it because of an even greater fear of humiliation. Whereas previous scenarios were about loss of control, this is about compromise and compromise can indeed be humiliating.

**How to Make It Good:** Don't just role play in the session…take it outside the office. Send an email message (always secure and private so no one will accidentally intercept!) or a handwritten letter with the "proof". Use aliases and pretend not to know each other. Converse about what the Dom is going to demand from the sub. The sub should object...but the Dom makes the threat. The more the innocent has to lose the better. So use your sick imagination as to whether she has children, a husband, or is a famous politician or movie star. She could also be a barely legal school girl.

**The Climax:** The sub goes through with the sexual demands, but negotiates for the end of the relationship if she does everything on the contract. However, the Dom lies and keeps on demanding sexual favors in return for his silence. He may even taunt her, forcing her to betray family and friends (cancel plans or rearrange schedule) just for his own amusement.

**Props:** For double the thrill video tape the sex or take photos. This creates more evidence to further blackmail the sub.

**Where?:** It may end in the bedroom but the journey and communication is citywide. You could even meet in a public place to discuss the "contract" for the first time.

**Variant:** A gangster could come to collects a debt from one sub and then take the debt from another sub, as in taking a husband's wife as collateral.

## 31. The Doctor's Examination

**The Setting:** The Doctor is now seeing his patient for healing, therapy and relief. Of course, since the patient is strapped in, she really can't object to whatever tests the doctor orders. The doctor has strapped the unsuspecting patient/victim in tightly and can now play with her with a wide arsenal of toys and other torture devices.

**Why It Works:** A Doctor is one of the most trusted professionals you ever meet so the idea of a perverted doctor toying with a helpless patient is disturbing and yet highly erotic for the patient, who both trusts the authority figure and yet feels violated by the treatment.

**How to Make It Good:** Don't make it too over the top "sexy". Make the doctor sound convincing and make the patient suspicious about what's going on. She thinks this is just a gynecological exam but he is ordering some strange tests and insists on testing all of her physical and sensual reflexes.

**The Climax:** The patient feels violated but by the end of it, she is strapped down and helpless to resist. All she can do is orgasm at his command, against her will, but enjoying every minute of the malpractice coercion.

**Props:** It's best to have either a strap down chair or at least some kind of restraint, since helplessness is what brings out fight or flight response. Make her strip and then tie her down tightly with no room to budge. Examine all of her sexual organs and then break out the dildos, vibrators, nipple clamps and clit ticklers.

**Where?:** Preferably a hotel, rented office, or even a man cave or storage room with minimal lighting.

**Variant:** A female doctor can take advantage of a male patient, or a nurse, in the same way.

**Multiples:** A doctor and his other Dom/sub nurse can torture the sub together.

## 32. The Dentist and the Patient

**The Setting:** You can guess the difference...whereas the Doctor keeps the patient awake for an exam, the dentist puts the patient to sleep. And then takes advantage of the patient sexually. The Dentist puts them to sleep with anesthesia and then takes the patient's clothes off, followed by sex or foreplay. The patient has no idea (or pretends not to know) what's happening.

**Why It Works:** The idea of being violated and yet not even knowing it is another lesson in guilt and sexual inhibition; while the Dentist Dom gets the opportunity to act on a taboo fantasy of rape play while the person sleeps. Of course this is illegal and immoral in real life, but a partner pretending to be asleep can allow you the fantasy with consent.

**How to Make It Good:** The partner should be completely quiet and preferably immobilized so that she can't squirm as if awake. This is also a good opportunity to use restraints of some sort.

**The Climax:** Afterward, the dentist suits up, unfastens restraints, hides all toys, and then puts the clothes back on the patient. He pretends that everything is fine. She has no idea what happened and thanks the dentist.

**Props:** A tie down table works best, but you can also use a bed, desk, flat couch, etc.

**Where?:** Preferably an office environment or at least a hotel.

**Variant:** Since consent is consent, if your partner is willing you can play with her while she actually sleeps. Toy with her breasts and vagina, slowly and gently, just avoiding waking her up. See how long you can go and then finish when she wakes up excited.

**Multiples:** A doctor and his other Dom/sub nurse can torture the sub together.

### 33. The Murderer and the Victim

**The Setting:** Warning: This is a very intense game and should not be tried until you've established good trust between each other as equal partners. This is not for all tastes. In this scenario, the Dom is torturing the victim. The idea that he's killed men/women before, makes the sub fear him and cooperate. However, the Murderer is not just sexually torturing her…he is slowly taking one sense away from her at a time. He kidnaps her, restrains her, and then blindfolds and ear-muffs her until she cannot see or hear.

**Why It Works:** Not only does this have the fear of a rape play and a dangerous man calling the action, but it also takes advantage of blind and deaf play. Once you remove your sense of sight and sound as a sub, you will feel the orgasmic sensations more intensely.

**How to Make It Good:** The murderer should be quiet while the victim pleads for her life. His silence will be scary, leading to an adrenaline rush, which will be heightened by foreplay and vibrator/dildo play. Electroshock is another game that can enhance the experience.

**The Climax:** The sub orgasms and then the Dom Murderer decides if she "lives" or "dies" (not real death, of course). Blood capsules or cutting could even be introduced at the end. This is not for all tastes, but for anyone that has a death or injury fetish it might be something to experiment with.

**Props:** Use firm rope, cuffs or bondage restraints. A ball gag if preferred, as well as a blindfold, and ear muffs or plugs to cut off hearing. You can have her wear headphones and listen to white noise which will alter her sense of hearing. If you really want to get imaginative cut off her sense of smell and taste by forcing her to taste something (like a ball gag) or smell something (perfume or another pleasant/unpleasant smell). Removing all of her senses will only heighten her sense of touch as the Dom tortures-pleasures her.

**Where?:** Preferably a hotel room.

**Variant:** If the murder scenario gets too disturbing, then do the same play with a Master of Martial Arts, who decides to remove a student's sight and sound so as to enhance their other reflexes.

**Multiples:** A doctor and his other Dom/sub nurse can torture the sub together.

## 34. The Trophy Spouse

**The Setting:** The Rich billionaire Dom decides to lend his wife/girlfriend to another person. He has noticed that his obedient wife seems attracted to his friend, or to a co-worker. But she is embarrassed and afraid when she is caught. Therefore, The Dom punishes her by giving her body to the friend, with full permission to him to do whatever he wants to her. She is afraid and shy but now the friend owns her for the night. Little did she know that the friend was a pervert of the highest order!

**Why It Works:** This is a conservative way of experimenting with polyamory without actually going that far in real life. A lot of monogamous women (and men) fantasize about being with someone else, but fear and love hold them back. Therefore, the idea of being "forced" to confront that attraction is a taboo idea. Whereas most couples are so jealous they never speak of temptations outside the relationship, in this game play, the couple uses that taboo to make for vivid sexual fantasy.

**How to Make It Good:** In this setting, the Dom can either assume the role of the Friend and change his personality, or he can be the Dom and tell her a vivid fantasy about the friend having rough sex with her. It always works better when you use a real person's name and character during the act.

**The Climax:** The friend (or more specifically the Dom pretending the friend is active) brings her to climax. The Dom warns her not to let such attraction show again or else he will give her body to the next person.

**Props:** Cuffing or restraining her works well, with the idea of the Friend exercising full control over her, not giving her a choice to say no.

**Where?:** Home is fine.

**Variant:** You can also make it a threesome by the Dom using an anal toy or extra dildo for double penetration.

**Multiples:** Make it a threesome in real life with a friend/acquaintance.

### 35. The Master and the Cuckold Couple

**The Setting:** The Master enjoys humiliating other men as well as women during his rough sex routine. Therefore, he chooses a wife or a girlfriend and makes violent love to her in front of her significant other. This is not actually a group sex game but can be done with just two partners with imaginative description. The cuckold is the "innocent" party who has no choice but to watch the Dom control his partner. He gives her an explicit fantasy describing what's happening.

**Why It Works:** This allows you both to toy with threesome fun in a safe setting. The Dom simply paints the fantasy of what is happening while pleasuring the sub, allowing her to visualize the humiliation of her husband while the Dom destroys and defiles her body for his own selfish pleasure.

**How to Make It Good:** Definitely use a blindfold so she can better visualize the scene happening. For the best results use real names of people you know, or if that's too uncomfortable, fictional characters or movie stars. This helps the visuals immensely. The Dom can give the sub her choice: either He is fucking her or a New Dom is fucking her in front of her (real life) husband.

**The Climax:** The Dom usually uses the cuckold as human furniture, humiliating him for as he has sex with the wife. In a bisexual scenario, he has sex with both of them.

**Props:** Restraints or cuffs might also help to enhance the sensations.

**Where?:** Anywhere.

**Variant:** Instead of a wife or girlfriend, you can experiment with family play. The Dom can be having sex with someone's mother or sister while a relative is forced to watch.

**Multiples:** A third party watches. If you don't actually want to cheat, the third party could pretend to be the innocent husband.

## 36. The Cuckold Husband, His Wife and Her Dom

**The Setting:** Not only can the female Domme reverse this cuckold scenario but she can also experiment with the point of view change. The man can play the cuckold and the woman can enjoy the feeling of cheating on her husband/boyfriend. This is not for all tastes but if partners are aroused by the idea you may find this a kinky scenario worth trying at least once. The woman gets all the pleasure and will either tell the cuckold husband how good the Dom is rough-housing her or she can have the cuckold male sub describe the scenario.

**Why It Works:** This is only two-partner play, and uses imagination. The wife gets to feel like the one in charge, describing her selfish pleasure, and the cuckold absorbs the humiliation. It's a safe way of experimenting in a game that you might never play in real life.

**How to Make It Good:** Use someone's real name, whether a person you know, or at least a movie star or fictional character. The woman berates the cuckold, explaining to him why she's cheating on him and why she is entitled to do so. If the cuckold is telling the story, he should express outrage and shock but also explain that he is helpless and knows he cannot persuade his wife to change her mind. Nor can he compete with the Dom so he accepts. He may even want his wife to be happy and so helps the Dom do a better job.

**The Climax:** The Dom finishes and makes a mess, usually all over the cuckold as well.

**Props:** Restraints and blindfold to heighten the experience.

**Where?:** Anywhere. Or the next time you're house sitting for a friend, work them into the scenario…only if they're hot, of course.

**Variant:** The cuckold wife would be a variant of this.

**Multiples:** A third party watches. If you don't actually want to cheat, the third party could pretend to be the innocent husband.

## 37. She Chooses Her Own Punishment

**The Setting:** The Dom has decided to punish the sub severely. But he knew in advance that she would be the one most qualified to come up with punishments. He made her make up the punishments (while aroused), the cards, and then put them into a hat. Then the next time he punished her, he made her choose one of her own punishments from the hat.

**Why It Works:** The anticipation factor works here. The Master ensures that the sub / slave is writing the worst punishments she can possibly bear. If she's good, she doesn't have to do them. That's the excuse she needs to write some good ideas. But she never expects she'll be punished and be made to do them.

**How to Make It Good:** Have her think up a number of punishments, such as no permission to orgasm for a set period of time, spanking, wearing nipple clamps, edging (almost orgasming but stopping suddenly and not finishing), ice or heat play, bondage and so on.

**The Climax:** The Dom finishes and consoles the bad sub.

**Props:** Have the sub create flash cards.

**Where?:** Anywhere.

**Variant:** Make a reward box as well as a punishment box. You can also create a marble game, where she draws good or bad marbles to signify reward or punishment. This is randomizing her punishment, therefore giving her the gift of anticipation. Teach her to fear the black marble and love the white marble.

**Multiples:** One Dom could create the punishments, or another sub, while another Dom presides. Or the Dom can have both subs choose cards.

### 38. The List From Hell!

**The Setting:** The Dom has decided to ask the sub for a re-clarification of what she is willing to do or not do. However, he has made his own list of questions, challenging her soft limits, and has denied her the privilege of knowing what they are. Therefore, he just asks YES or NO to a number of numbers. She answers by her instinct. Then he tells her what she agreed to do.

**Why It Works:** The anticipation is intense and once she realizes that she "agreed" to being defiled, a rush of adrenaline hits her.

Whereas most BDSM contracts are negotiated explicitly (and yes, hard limits must always be respected) one fun way to toy with the feelings of comfort is to contractually obligate the sub to do whatever is written on the secret list.

**How to Make It Good:** Since this is still a two-player scene, and since you cannot exploit her "hard limits," think of compromises that would allow her to "do" the task, to a reasonable degree without going too far over her personal limits. For example, a threesome scenario might be a hard limit, but fantasizing about it could be a soft limit she is willing to do. If she says no to anal sex, then one list item could be anal stimulation without intercourse.

**The Climax:** The sub compromises and fulfills the activity.

**Props:** Depending on the question.

**Where?:** Anywhere

**Variant:** Instead of yes or no, you can have her pick Multiple Choice questions. This might include confusing "answers" she has to choose from (without knowing the question). Once she understands the question she is horrified at what she has agreed to!

## 39. The Mugger and the Victim

**The Setting:** The mugger doesn't have much. All he brought with him was a knife. But when he sees the beautiful sub Victim walking by, he decides to kidnap her and threaten her with a knife. He takes her somewhere private and then tears her clothes off with his knife.

**Why It Works:** A knife is scary! Whereas you may have experimented with a fake gun in other scenarios, knives have the bonus of being prickly to the skin. Experiment with rape play and introduce her to knife play at the same time.

**How to Make It Good:** The knife should be chilled for even more sensual sensation when touching the skin. Be careful not to cut the sub, unless she wants it.

**The Climax:** All of her clothes are torn to shreds and sex commences.

**Props:** A knife. Learn how to use it and the best way to cut through clothing. Away from the skin! A blindfold can also enhance the sensation and make the sub believe you are cutting her when you're not.

**Where?:** Anywhere.

**Variant:** You can also use a fake gun or a whip if you're afraid of accidentally cutting her.

## 40. Truth or Dare Date

**The Setting:** This is a Dom taking his sub out on a date...the usual rules of no talking to anyone else and being subservient. But with one exception. The Dom demands the sub answer all Truth questions. If she lies, the Dom forces her to do a dare. The sub answers his questions but the Dom declares that she is lying. He makes her perform degrading acts, not in public, but in private public.

**Why It Works:** The sub's arousal comes from the fact that she is quiet and cannot publicly refuse anything he requests. Nobody else catches wise but she is aroused and so has paranoid thoughts of other people staring at her.

**How to Make It Good:** The Dom teases her as the night goes on, demanding her to remove her underwear in the ladies room. Or to masturbate in a private location. Or he secretly touches her under the table or fondles her in a darkened movie theater. Or he passes erotic notes telling her what he's going to do later.

**The Climax:** After a night of teasing the Dom has sex with her, but also brainwashes her into admitting that what she knows is "true" is actually a lie. She confesses to whatever truth he drags out of her.

**Where?:** At a restaurant or theater.

**Variant:** He can humiliate the sub further by demanding she embarrass herself in public, not erotically, but doing strange things or funny things.

**Multiples:** If both are game, take the sub to an erotic theater or swinger party where he can embarrass her out in public sexually.

## 41. Secret Toy Shared

**The Setting:** The Dom further humiliates the sub by forcing her to wear a vibrator out in public while he watches. This special hidden vibrator may even be radio controlled by the Dom. He gives her no warning but may activate it on the phone, or when she's ordering food or talking to an old friend.

**Why It Works:** It's a great form of humiliation as well as reluctant arousal. She surrenders all control to him but must also control her own passion from embarrassing herself. The Dom can even follow her around for a few hours and torture her from a distance in secret.

**How to Make It Good:** Do not allow the sub to have sex or masturbate for a long while before the hidden vibrator stimulation begins. By the end of the game she will be begging for release.

**The Climax:** The sub cannot orgasm until the Dom gives permission.

**Props:** A radio controlled vibrator that attached onto the sub.

**Where?:** Anywhere.

**Variant:** If you two don't venture out in public much, the Dom can force the sub to make phone calls and risk humiliation that way. The male sub version of this game can also be benefited by taking Viagra or another natural aphrodisiac in advance of going out. He will be hard and horny but unable to come unless given permission.

**Multiples:** The Dom can arrange in secret for a friend to talk to the sub for an extended period of time. The sub is highly aroused and the Friend pretends to be oblivious but keeps her for a long time talking. The sub can't seem to leave the conversation. Eventually, the friend may let her on the secret by saying sexual things.

### 42. Human Sex Doll

**The Setting:** The Dom wants his own human sex doll so he removes the right of the sub to move on her own or talk. She is just to stand or sit where he puts her and say nothing. He can move her arms or legs however she wants. She remains passive, even when he strips her, dresses her and has sex with her.

**Why It Works:** This can be humiliating as well as painful if restraints, rope or cuffs are used.

**How to Make It Good:** Half the fun is in exploration. The Dom explores the sub's body and all of her orifices, touching and probing wherever he wants. He can also torture her nipples, vagina or butt.

**The Climax:** The sub must allow him to continue until climax but she is forbidden to make a sound or show any response. If she fails, she will be punished.

**Props:** The Dom should dress up the sub in whatever sexy clothing he wants, treating her like a Barbie doll. He must dress her since she cannot move.

**Where?:** Anywhere.

**Variant:** Add another layer of fun by allowing the sub to talk and object, but still being unable to move or stop the Dom. Maybe she is under a magic spell or mind control and frozen in place.

**Multiples:** The Dom can move two subs around and make them simulate sex with each other.

### 43. The Dom Brands the Sub

**The Setting:** The Dom decides to write on the sub's body for his own amusement. He draws on her body in paint and takes video or photos of what he wrote. The words are usually dirty, such as "slut, whore, used by \_\_\_," and so on. Or the Dom may choose to put "property of" on the sub's body.

**Why It Works:** This is a more dramatic example of dirty talking. The partner's body is his canvas and since all the paint comes off he can use his imagination. The Dom can even instruct the sub to write his words on her own body.

**How to Make It Good:** The marking goes across the partner's chest or breasts, or on her butt, or above the vagina. Somewhere intimate. In addition to words, the Dom can also write what he is going to do to the sub.

**The Climax:** The Dom can wait until sex is over and the sub is sweaty and messy to write. Or he could hide the words from the sub until they both finish and then she can read them.

**Props:** Magic markers or edible safe body paint.

**Where?:** Take the sub to a public place and tell her to write on her body in secret in the bathroom and take a photo of it.

**Variant:** The Dom can eventually require that the words be permanent, such as the sub wearing the words in secret to work. Or he could brand (burn) her or tattoo the words permanently as a sign of ownership.

**Multiples:** Tell other people and show them the brand symbol / ownership. A collar can be used instead of a tattoo. The sub will be proud to show her proof of ownership to a stranger or to another Dom or sub.

## 44. Sexual Brainwashing 101

**The Setting:** The new Dom has dropped off the sub at a farm where she will be reeducated to be trained slut. The new Dom will be breaking in the sub and teaching her not just how to behave but how to unconsciously respond to Dom's actions and words without request. This works by associate sexual response with either a word, a sound or an action. The Dom will subconsciously train her to get horny, involuntarily.

**Why It Works:** Training is half punishment but half hypnotic commands. The Farm Dom trains the sub through consistent speaking, taking his time and explaining in great detail what will happen in the future. He will explain sexual techniques he will do and the other Dom will do and then describe them in vivid detail. He will order the partner to beg for it, anticipate it until they literally FEEL it.

**How to Make It Good:** Associate her maximum state of arousal with a chosen word, a name or a physical action—like grabbing her wrist or something small. This way, after some time you can program that as an anchor and force her to feel aroused later on, upon command, and wherever or whenever. You can do the same thing with a piece of jewelry by forcing her to wear it during maximum state of arousal or even to wear a bell or chime so that they associate that specific noise with sex.

**The Climax:** The Dom will eventually train the sub to be obedient to the anchor word or object, and deliver her back to the other Dom trained. The most fun will be turning her on in public and causing embarrassment and reluctant arousal.

**Props:** It can be anything but consistency is the key.

**Where?:** Anywhere.

**Variant:** Any sexual fetish can take the place of sex for this training. For example, some subs enjoy breast and lactation play and so will have the scenario of the farmer milking them as if a cow. They will learn to associate certain stimuli with breastfeeding arousal.

**Multiples:** One Dom can give the sub to a Second Dom for training and then take her back with the new behavior.

Releasing Your Inhibitions: Pain/Pleasure Tolerance

These activities are for extreme highs and adrenaline rushes but necessarily sexual acts. That means you can try them with a Dom/Sub who doesn't want sex or who wants to try something more intense than just sex—such as pleasure and pain training.

## 45. The Exorcist and Demon Girl

**The Setting:** An exorcist must try to rid the girl of the demon. The Demon is making her do inappropriate things and usually provocative that is opposite to the sub's nature. The exorcist is inexperienced but must press on anyway and rid the girl of the evil spirit. Along the way though, the sub will be forced to do what she fears the most. (Soft limit activities)

**Why It Works:** This is a good dynamic to think outside of just sexual relations and challenge the sub with soft limits by relieving her of responsibility, her fear, by letting the Demon take over her. For example, if the sub likes the idea of swearing but is too shy to try it, the "demon" could possess her and start swearing. If the sub is too shy to sing or to belly dance in public, but really wants to do it, the possession act can help her feel the excitement of doing it, without the responsibility.

**How to Make It Good:** Choose soft limit activity that she's ordinarily afraid to try. This is also very good for people who are religious, were religious in the past, or have a special fetish for religious scenarios.

**The Climax:** The demon is possessed and the sub gets to do something that she's always been afraid to do.

**Props:** Restraints work since the demon must be restrained for protection. A demon mask might also help the sub feel uninhibited.

**Where?:** Anywhere

**Variant:** The Dom could actually assume the role of the demon possessed boy, if necessary, and the sub can be the clergy; this way, the Dom can help show the sub how to indulge in that forbidden or taboo behavior she likes but is too shy to enjoy.

**Multiples:** Two priests can preside over the demon possessed girl, torturing her as a means to get the demon out.

## 46. The Deprogrammer and Cult Follower

**The Setting:** The sub is a brainwash victim escaping a cult. The Dom is the deprogrammer. Depending on your personal taste, you can be an evil deprogrammer or an objective deprogrammer. But the intent is to train the sub to be a new person. The sub is confused and vulnerable. The Dom can teach her new moral codes, new ethics and new trains of thought.

**Why It Works:** The Dom gets full authority to reprogram her to change her thinking and behavior. This can be used for therapeutic reasons; as in helping to boost her self-esteem or even for mind-warping purposes; getting angry whenever someone uses the word "late." Thinking that they're an animal or an opposite sex gender.

**How to Make It Good:** Much of the reprogramming process is hypnotic commands (usually read while the subject lies down and loses consciousness) or falls asleep. They will still hear the commands even when under.

**The Climax:** Of course, the one thing cult programming and deprogramming have in common is the "discipline" process. Therefore, besides hypnotic training, related to soft limits, the other part of this task is designing painful punishments that will teach the sub to fear certain thought patterns or impulsive actions that the Dom wants to get rid of.

**Props:** Using strong visuals, including "anchor" objects is very powerful for associations. For example, a watch or a piece of jewelry.

**Where?:** Anywhere.

**Variant:** Another variant might be instead of deprogrammer, a psychiatrist or psychologist that takes advantage of his patients by training them to do strange and unnatural things for his own sense of pleasure.

**Multiples:** The Dom can delegate authority to a Second Dom for training.

## 47. Mad Scientist and Subject

**The Setting:** A mad scientist has strapped down a victim / subject and is performing non-sexual but still bizarre research. He is evil and dominant while the sub is helpless. What these experimental activities are could be anything from spanking to tying up and binding, ice / heat play, or tickling. The Dom's intent is to see how far he can push the sub in terms of torture and release. This is ideal for subspace game play.

**Why It Works:** The sub is restrained, either in a doctor's chair or flat board or even a bed. Something that renders them helpless and completely subservient to the scientist, who tests their endurance.

**How to Make It Good:** Remove as many senses as possible, including sight with a blindfold, hearing with headphones and white music, and if you desire, a ball gag or strong neutral scent that is overwhelming. This will cause her to focus on the experiments you do.

**The Climax:** She will feel a rush of adrenaline as you edge her and increase the pain, only to bring it down and then back up again. Although sex isn't necessary, she could easily be brought to orgasm if you both want that.

**Props:** Restraints, rope, blind fold, earphones.

**Where?:** Anywhere

**Variant:** Sexual pain, such as nipple clamps, chastity belts or anal beads or plugs could be used for semi-sexual torture but not overt sexual intercourse.

**Multiples:** The Scientist can have a Dom or sub assist them in torturing the sub. Such as, holding instruments or actually using one torture tool while the Dom uses another.

### 48. The Hypnotist and the Client

**The Setting:** The hypnotist "puts the patient to sleep" although she doesn't literally have to fall asleep for this experiment. The Dom then gives her hypnotic commands not related to sex but related to life change.

**Why It Works:** This is like the deprogramming exercise, except that the hypnotist uses only hypnotic commands and doesn't put as much emphasis on physical punishment. However, he may subject her to mental punishment, in the way of negative associations with certain words, though patterns and so on. He trains her subconscious mind to reject thoughts because of negative imagery, feelings or physical reactions he creates.

**How to Make It Good:** The Dom should write out the script in advance and practice delivering the lines slowly and with proper pronunciation. Remember as the Dom to paint yourself as the strong visual that she concentrates on, the center of all positive emotion.

**The Climax:** The Dom subjects her to her soft limit, surpassing boundaries only when she's ready and has been hypnotized into.

**Props:** Blindfold works wonders.

**Where?:** Anywhere.

**Variant:** The hypnosis can spread beyond the session and into the sub's away life. The Dom programs her to do homework and fulfill a lists of task in relation to his long-term goal of changing her.

## 49. Mummification and Sacrifice

**The Setting:** The Dom ties up the sub, preparing her for burial. She may be "dead" or alive, but she cannot move either way. He ties her up so snug she can't move. She cannot speak either. She may send him messages with her eyes, letting him know she's still alive but she cannot speak. After she's mummified the Dom can play with her body, subjecting her to ice play or knifes. Spanking and pinching will also feel much more intense, as there is no rope to worry about.

**Why It Works:** Her inability to speak, either voluntary or gagged shut, makes her feel especially vulnerable.

**How to Make It Good:** For more ambiance, make it more of a religious or esoteric / magic ritual. Half the fun and adrenaline will be the sub's unfamiliarity with what is happening. She knows that you will respect her soft and hard limits, but she doesn't understand the ritual aspect of her mummification and sacrifice. This will cause anticipation. Mumble chants or have music playing as she wrapped up.

**The Climax:** The mummy is taken, sacrificed (played with) and "buried." When the scene ends she is cut loose. Remember though to either have a safe word or signal. And if you are the Dom, you should check the sub's temperature and behavior anyway, as there is a slight risk of overheating, especially if you don't ask for confirmation that she's still conscious and feeling awake.

**Props:** Saran wrap is an alternative to the other restraints and is the best and cheapest way to mummify a sub. They are usually nude when the wrapping begins. Make the scene exciting with relics, Gothic décor, scary music, masks, and the like.

**Where?:** Anywhere

**Variant:** Hog tied by a cowboy, strapped down by a Nazi scientist, kidnapped by a drug lord, the endless scenarios are always fun.

**Multiples:** The Dom can delegate authority to a second Dom or sub; one to mummify the other to touch and play with, or shared between both. She could even be passed around to a group of Doms who can all take part in playing with her once she is tied up.

### 50. Character Playing (Non Erotic)

**The Setting:** This is a somewhat complicated exercise in which the Dom assumes the role of a real life person in the past of the sub. This is not sexual but is helpful in letting go of baggage, old demons and ill feelings about the past. The Dom plays the part of the person the sub resents. She says what she wants to say to that person, to the Dom. Instead of punishing the sub, the Dom simply listens and reacts. He may ask forgiveness or may taunt her, depending on what the sub thinks the real person would do.

**Why It Works:** This is not really a game but a cathartic exercise. Sometimes in life the sub can never really get closure with a long lost person who wronged them. This is the next best thing.

**How to Make It Good:** Be very specific and realistic in what that other person would say. The sub may become angry or cry, but the Dom will always listen and react naturally.

NOTE: If the past involves abuse, the sub should think about seeing a therapist before the Dom gets involved. Seeing a therapist and talking her feelings out first, will help her better process her feelings. Otherwise, she may lash out at the Dom and become very upset, leading to more trauma.

**The Climax:** After the scene, the Dom will comfort the sub in real life, explaining how the process will help her to move on.

**Where?:** Anywhere, maybe even in a place where the sub and the original person first met.

**Multiples:** If you like the idea but don't feel comfortable pretending to be someone else, as a Dom, then consider meeting another Dom and exchanging or swapping subs just for the new experiences. This is an alternative to changing your own natural personality as a Dom.

## 51. Becoming Someone Else

**The Setting:** In this scenario, both Dom and sub assume different identities but the trick is they take it to the outside world. They become new characters by meeting new friends, doing new activities and ingratiating themselves in the lifestyle. Then they meet a second time, acting opposite characters, and enjoy activity on a new level.

**Why It Works:** Blending their new identities into the real world around them makes this more interesting. The Dom can speak to the sub around other people who are oblivious as to what is happening but noticing the conversation.

**How to Make It Good:** The sub is opposite the usual sub so she can throw curveballs at the Dom and say No. This may seem contrary, but remember this is opposites day. The Dom must now figure out how to break the sub using charm, and eventually punishment and training.

**The Climax:** The Dom is persuading the tough sub that only he can punish her the right way. The sub must decide if she likes him in this character. He may have to adopt opposite personality traits, and reward/punishment but that's what the sub will like. Falling into the hands of a new master and learning new training.

**Where?:** Out in public for the start and then private locations for the punishment.

**Variant:** This can be sexual or nonsexual. After the first encounter the sub / Dom can decide if this was a one-time experiment or if they want to keep seeing each other with these new identities.

# Conclusion

As you can see there are many games and scenes to choose from. Let your imagination go wild and add your own personal touch to each scene. Thanks for reading!

# Other Books by Elizabeth Cramer

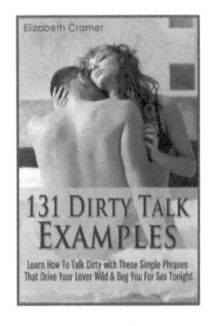

131 Dirty Talk Examples: Learn How To Talk Dirty with These Simple Phrases That Drive Your Lover Wild & Beg You For Sex Tonight

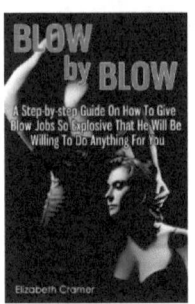

Blow By Blow - A Step-by-step Guide On How To Give Blow Jobs So Explosive That He Will Be Willing To Do Anything For You

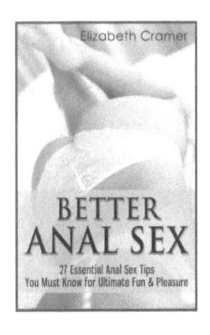

Better Anal Sex - 27 Essential Anal Sex Tips You Must Know for Ultimate Fun & Pleasure

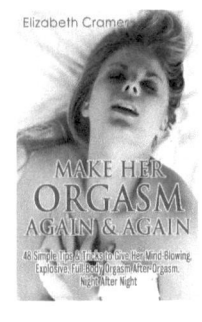

Make Her Orgasm Again and Again: 48 Simple Tips & Tricks to Give Her Mind-Blowing, Explosive, Full-Body Orgasm After Orgasm, Night After Night

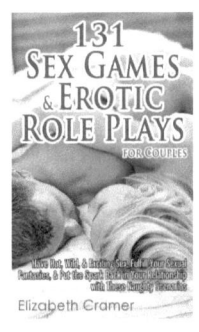

131 Sex Games & Erotic Role Plays for Couples: Have Hot, Wild, & Exciting Sex, Fulfill Your Sexual Fantasies, & Put the Spark Back in Your Relationship with These Naughty Scenarios

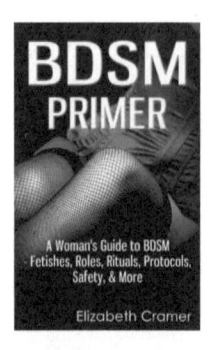

BDSM Primer - A Woman's Guide to BDSM - Fetishes, Roles, Rituals, Protocols, Safety, & More

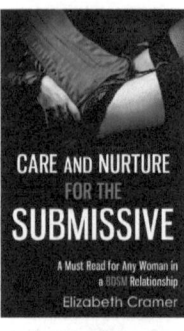

Care and Nurture for the Submissive - A Must Read for Any Woman in a BDSM Relationship

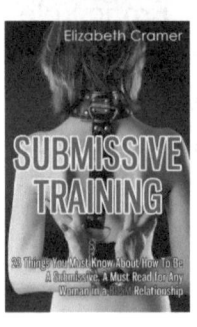

Submissive Training: 23 Things You Must Know About How To Be A Submissive. A Must Read For Any Woman In A BDSM Relationship

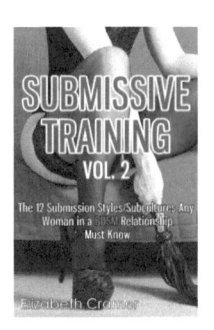

Submissive Training Vol. 2: The 12 Submission Styles/Subcultures Any Woman In A BDSM Relationship Must Know

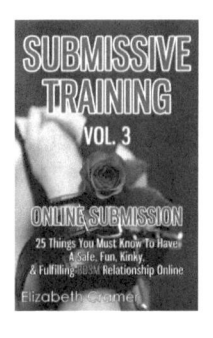

Submissive Training Vol. 3: Online Submission - 25 Things You Must Know To Have A Safe, Fun, Kinky, & Fulfilling BDSM Relationship Online

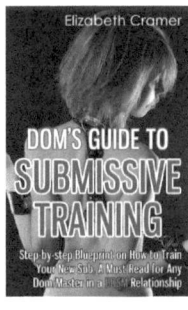

Dom's Guide To Submissive Training: Step-by-step Blueprint On How To Train Your New Sub. A Must Read For Any Dom/Master In A BDSM Relationship

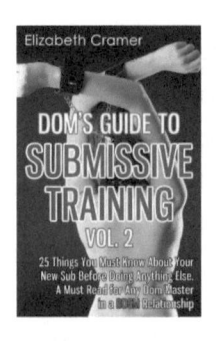

Dom's Guide To Submissive Training Vol. 2: 25 Things You Must Know About Your New Sub Before Doing Anything Else. A Must Read For Any Dom/Master In A BDSM Relationship

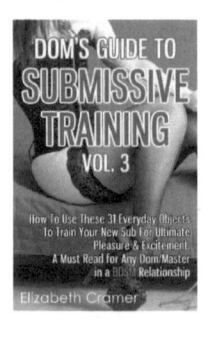

Dom's Guide To Submissive Training Vol. 3: How To Use These 31 Everyday Objects To Train Your New Sub For Ultimate Pleasure & Excitement. A Must Read For Any Dom/Master In A BDSM Relationship

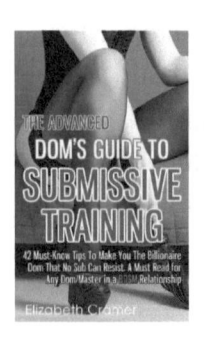

The Advanced Dom's Guide To Submissive Training: 42 Must-Know Tips To Make You The Billionaire DOM That No Sub Can Resist. A Must Read For Any Dom/Master In A BDSM Relationship

Made in United States
Troutdale, OR
02/27/2024

18030016R00066